Trip to Fitness

A Fitness Preparation Guide to Making a New You

BEATRICE O. SARGIN

ISBN: 978-1-4834-8965-0 (sc)
ISBN: 978-1-4834-8964-3 (e)

Lulu Publishing Services rev. date: 08/06/2018

Dedication

This book is dedicated to the loving memory of

Aaliyah D. Haughton (1979 – 2001).

Contents

Acknowledgements

I want to appreciate my family for their support in writing this book. My parents Mr. Luke & Mrs. Beatrice Ezeighu, my siblings Anthony Sargin, Paul Sargin, Mrs. Gertrude & Mr. Stephen Udofia, Mrs. Juliet Sargin and the rest of my family members. Thank you all for your rich love and support all through this project.

MESSAGE FROM THE AUTHOR

This book provides the reader with quick and easy reference to information which is required to guide you in your fitness trip. This book is not exhaustive; it attempts to include information that will guide you adequately to make the right choices to get the best of your fitness results hoped for. Ensure to consult with your physician to give you a comprehensive break down on your health status before beginning any Fitness trip.

This book is subject to periodic review and can be updated over time.

Beatrice Sargin

Author

Preparation

When an individual has a perception of themselves becoming fit, an anchor that binds their body, mind and soul is formed. When this happens, they tend to send a positive signal that relates simultaneously to the law of attraction which connects their positive energy to their focus power. As we all know, fitness always comes to mind, but the ability to fight those negative energies and signal to achieve our desired fitness purpose makes you the winner. It is easier to say "I Want to Be Fit", on the other hand, to do what it takes makes you your own Hero. You have to do what it takes from the point of the decision making to your trip to fitness. It takes a stronger positive energy to work extremely hard to bring this perception into reality. Fitness then becomes a burning passionate desire that overwhelms an individual as their shadow when it comes to actualization. Fitness is HARD; there are no smooth fitness journeys. If it were easy, everyone will do it with a snap, but the nature of the HARDNESS makes it adventurous and Great.

Have you made up your mind yet? There are some tips to help you get prepared for this fitness trip to stay healthy and catch the fit train before it leaves again. People often miss their fitness train due to their busy schedules, lack of focus due to distractions and uncertainty by asking the wrong questions, hence wasting more time than to keep up with their workout routines resulting in setbacks and final withdrawal.

The time has come to get up and go ahead. You have your cool new exercise equip, your special new claim to fame exercise shoes. Truth be told, all your new apparatus is arranged and prepared to go. Presently you are prepared to go ahead… right?

One moment. A little preparation tip goes far.

Fitness is an "I" element, which means everything depends on your decisions and efforts from start to finish. There are mistakes that are made across the line due to asking the wrong questions. Some distractive question Individuals regularly ask include: **"How can I lose weight?"** or **"What is the best or fastest approach to get in shape?"** Everyone wants to get in shape VERY FAST so they tend to ask popular FAQs as such whose complete answers you can't easily find on Google search engines but fragments instead of asking the right questions. If you've been asking those questions, you are just 30 percent (%) ready to be fit as it shows just that you are not ready for the fitness adventures. The question often ignored is one that is similarly as imperative and pertinent in your fitness trip which is: **"How can I best be prepared to get the most out of my workout(s)?"** PERFECT!

The response to this inquiry is, obviously, an extremely individualized reaction which relies upon a huge number of components. For example, the physical profile of the individual asking **"How old are you? How is your general well being?** etc. the exercise they have arranged, the level of wellness effectively achieved and the measure of involvement with the action of the game arranged.

There are some DOs & TRY NOT that are vital things to do after answering the perfect question above before any other thing:

1. **DO** : Take pictures of your present status

Ø **Try Not To:** Freak out when you look at the picture and think of how long it will take you for the body you are about to build.

Nobody enjoys his or her Day 1 photographs or estimations. Yet, by catching the majority of the fundamental data (the amount you measure, how enormous your abdomen is, the thing that you look like shirtless or in a two-piece), you'll build up a beginning spot. At that point, when you bring down this data once more, you'll perceive the amount you've changed.

2. **DO:** Weigh yourself once per week.

Ø **Try Not To:** Weigh yourself consistently.

Your weight can change each day in light of how much sodium you devoured the day preceding, the amount you sweated amid your exercise, regardless of whether you went to the washroom, what time it is, and so on. In case you're the sort who could get debilitated from seeing your weight go up a pound or (at least two) in 24 hours. It'll give you a superior general feeling of the pattern your weight is heading in. Simply remember you may pick up a couple of pounds amid an initial couple of long stretches of starting a program.

3. **DO:** Eat for the body you need — NOT the body you have.

Ø **Try Not To:** Cut out the greater part of your most loved sustenance.

On the off chance that you truly need to be hopeless and set yourself up for dis-appointment, slice out all that you get a kick out of the chance to eat. Probably, your eating regimen is extremely awful, a great deal of stuff you like may need to go. Pop, broiled nourishment, super sugary espresso drinks… Think of this new adventure as a training camp. You're cultivating a habit for the body you've gen-erally desired. Hence, nourish that body with the sustenance it needs. Complex carbs, lean proteins, and heaps of supplement stuffed vegetables. The other 25% of the time, don't worry about it. On the off chance that you truly need that brew or that treat, have it. One treat or one lager won't be your destruction.

4. **DO:** Plan your dinners and sort out your kitchen.

Ø **Try Not To:** Make last minute dinner/meals decisions as this won't be of great assistance to you on this trip.

By arranging your dinners, you make it simpler to eat more advantageously on the grounds that you don't need to consider it consistently. You simply get your breakfast or potentially your lunch and go.

4

5. **DO:** Push through the soreness.

Ø **Try Not To:** Push yourself to the point of damage.

At whatever point, begin another workout schedule, accept to be sore for the initial two weeks. Endure the aches with hard work & perseverance. Regardless of whether the soreness doesn't keep going that long, it enables the brain to get in the correct zone. Soreness is a privilege of entry, yet it's as yet hard to manage. *Try not to* go 100% on Day One, and slope things up every day in light of how you feel. On the off chance that you do get sore, back off, however, **don't stop**. Completing an exercise at half is a great deal superior to nothing. It will likewise enable your soreness to blur faster.

6. **DO:** Expect to be somewhat eager and grouchy at first.

Ø **Try Not To:** Fall once again into old negative behaviour patterns.

Regardless of what transformation you're making — whether it's another wellness routine or a cross-country move — there will undoubtedly be developing agonies. Change is awkward. Get ready to get a handle on a tad bit of sorts — you may be eager, you may feel sore, you may be somewhat surly accordingly — and it's more probable you'll have a simpler progress into your new way of life. *Soreness and craving go as one.* When you're sore, you're separated and that affects yearning to repair your body. They'll die down together. To speed things up, consider focusing on nourishment or supplementation. The correct sustenance and the ideal time will limit your want to overeat.

7.   **DO:** Have a realistic plan and follow your exercise schedule.

Ø **Try Not To:** Don't hold up until Monday to begin again on the off chance that you miss an exercise.

In the event that you missed an exercise in light of infection or travel or you simply didn't have a craving for doing it, don't stress. Simply hit it up to make up for the time loss!

8.   **DO:** Schedule your calendar to set out enough time for training. Get back on the program in the event that you tumble off.

Ø **Try Not To:** Don't pummel yourself, feel like you've fizzled, or hold up until the following day/week/month to begin once again.

Nobody is great. Not me, not you, and not our coaches. Everybody has an undesirable dinner now and then or misses an exercise. Try not to give that a chance to characterize your day, your week, or your month. Simply get ideal back on track. You're on an excursion and en route, there will be a couple of misses. In the event that you lift yourself appropriate move down and continue onward, you'll arrive there eventually.

9.   **DO:** Share what you're doing and discover individuals who will keep you responsible.

Ø **Try Not To:** Listen to the haters.

In the event that you share what you're doing with people around you, there's a more prominent probability you'll succeed on the grounds that you're making a social-emotionally supportive network that you're responding to. There may be individuals who mock your trip, however, disregard them. They have their purposes behind doing as such (generally the reasons come from envy or dread), so simply remain positive and connect with your emotionally supportive network when you require help.

10. **DO:** Monitor your progress reports once in a while.

Ø **Try Not To:** Frequently compare yourself in shredding with a colleague on the trip.

No two people have the same body mechanism and there's a tendency that you might be in a program with a colleague or probably started training the same time. But the other person seems to be shedding more pounds faster than you. Don't punish yourself for it by being negative to yourself. Understand your body during the process. Keep tabs of your personal data progress reports and stay motivated on your fitness goals.

Get On The Fit Track

After getting acquainted with the DOs and TRY NOT in this fitness trip you've embarked on. Keep in mind that you must thoroughly understand the significance of the best possible warm-up and chill off, here are some other, maybe lesser known, tips for getting the most out of your fitness exercise:

- *Professional Personal Trainer*

Find a personal trainer to guide you through. Getting the go-ahead from your trainer is an essential initial step while leaving on another or sloped up wellness schedule. Call them and set up that physical exam you might not have had in a while. Keep in mind that you are grinding away, converse with your doctor about your foreseen wellness regimen. He or she knows your wellbeing status and knows you and may have some extra tips for you and your extremely singular wellbeing and wellness circumstance.

- **Brain Over Issue**

When you have all the fitting rigging and you get the all-unmistakable, mentally getting ready for the new challenge(s) can be an exceptionally compelling following up stage. This regularly incorporates reviewing your motivation for leaving on this street in any case, imagining your objectives and envisioning your coveted results. This is a fundamental piece of the exercise routine for a large number of the present best competitors.

- **Filling Up**

Some swear by the correct mix of supplements at particular time allotments prior and post-exercise while others don't eat at all prior and may even feel physically as well as rationally unfit to eat after also.

Both of the above is likely fine and dandy. In the event that you are a normal exerciser and work out a couple of times each week, you truly shouldn't be as worried about post-practice nourishments in light of the fact that your body will have enough time between exercises to recoup. Pre-practice nourishments happen to more significance in the event that you are not following an adjusted eating routine and are not taking in enough calories at general interims for the duration of the day. You may get hazard episodes of hypoglycaemia (low glucose) or you might be exhausted and not get the most out of your exercise.

If we are considering specificity:

On the off chance that you will eat before your exercise, it is for the most part savvy to do as such around 30 minutes to an hour earlier. The perfect pre-exercise feast is little and made out of complex sugars. Cases incorporate portions of an entire grain bagel or a bit of natural product.

After your exercise, hold up around 15 minutes- an hour to eat. Now, fit protein and complex sugar-rich nourishments are useful in supplanting exhausted glycogen stores in the muscles. Protein likewise helps repair muscles. A couple of cuts of turkey with some entire grain wafers or a glass of low-fat drain with a bit of natural product would both be impeccable alternatives.

- *Hydrate! Drink lots of water!*

Also, you've heard it earlier yet this truly is sufficiently critical to hear over and over:

Water is basic for ideal physical execution and general functions. Ensure that you are keeping yourself sufficiently hydrated some time recently, amid, and after your exercise regardless of whether you don't feel especially parched. Drink up and drink regularly. Presently, do what needs to be done to get your body sufficiently cleansed and stabilized.

- *Roll out little improvements.*

The greatest misstep individuals make and frequently why we tumble off the fleeting trend is on the grounds that we go too hard too early and attempt to change everything without a moment's delay. This isn't viable. Make simple, little changes every week to move towards your objectives. I generally advise my young men and ladies to roll out one improvement every week and continue conveying them over so they turn into a propensity. At that point, the following week that continues, In addition to you may evacuate handled sugars… et cetera.

- ***Try to move your body each day. No specific reasons required.***

Begin little, particularly on the off chance that you are new to wellness routine. It doesn't mean that you'll have to run a marathon consistently. What you need to do is influence a routine out of moving your body. Begin your day on a high with some invigorating endorphins. Begin with a basic walk every day, and then perhaps you increase it to 3 strolls and 2 rec centre classes and so on.

On the off chance that you neglect to set you up, get ready to come up short.

- ***Consistency is critical.***

Be consentient with preparing, slim down and your outlook and I guarantee results will be revealed.

- ***Slip-ups happen.***

We are generally humans, we as a whole have awful days; oversights and slip-ups are a characteristic piece of life. There is no point worrying about it. On the off chance that you foul up on your eating regimen or miss an instructional meeting, don't worry about it and rebuff yourself, simply get back on track straight away.

- ***Appreciate the voyage.***

Truly obviously the goal matters yet you Need TO appreciate the trip. In the event that you despise each moment of your new changes/way of life, it won't be a long haul and it isn't viable. On the off chance that you appreciate every last day, figuring out how to love the new sound sustenance, the way your body feels when you eat well, the endorphins of training and so forth then you will probably stick to your pattern and remain on track for the long run. I likewise recommend that you compensate progress. Maybe that implies a solid treat dinner each fortnight or a back rub since you've worked really hard. Reward the little wins since they matter. Little wins reliably make for extraordinary achievement.

Instructions On How To Prepare To Begin A Wellness Excursion

Most importantly, congrats on choosing to begin your wellness routine. How about going more than few stages that will assist you to begin? In the event that you are new to Fitness and wellness and you're hoping to better your way of life or are hoping to get back on track then this post is for you. The following are my best tips for beginning the fitness trip.

- Know that at in the first place, you will suck. The primary stationary bicycle session you finish? It will suck. The first occasion when you swim down the fitness focus pool and back? Suck. Your first lap you do around a track? Suck, suck, and suck. In any case, the imperative thing to know is that you will show signs of improvement. Also, the better thing? It won't take long.

On the off chance that you regard to manage your routines properly, you should begin seeing the change in up to **14 days.** Furthermore, after you get to where you can serenely do some cardio exercises for 30 or 45 minutes, you will begin enhancing considerably quicker.

- Beware of every one of your enticements in the form of cravings, whatever it may be for you. For example, potato chips, frozen yogurt, treats, chocolate, pop.

- Go shopping… purchase new foods grown from the ground, lean protein, nuts (as well as nut kinds of margarine) and complex starches (sweet potatoes, darker rice, quinoa)

- Tell your family/companions that you are working on getting yourself Fit… it will keep you more responsible.

- Take estimations (chest, midriff, hips, thighs and arms) and pictures (front and side view). You can likewise measure yourself, however, depending more on the measuring tape and pictures to keep tabs on your development.

- Take a wellness test. This will help you to get your pattern. At that point re-try this wellness test each month or somewhere in the vicinity and keep tabs on your development. You will do only 3 works out. Push-ups (test abdominal are a quality), jumping squats (test bring down body quality and cardiovascular wellness) and board (tests your centre quality) Set a clock for 1 minute and record what number of redundancies you can do in 1 minute.

- Start a nourishment diary and track your sustenance. This is very import-ant, it will help you to utilize your ideal meal plans properly and help you with an undistracted focus towards what you want.

- Get yourself geared up, whatever fitness kit you require and you know it will be beneficial for your fitness trip, get prepared.

- Keep an exercise diary (like a bullet journal) and track your exercises. Have a beginning stage and keep tabs on your development. This is the place everything starts. This is the place the procedure begins and you have chosen to roll out an improvement. The following advancement is a stand-out amongst other approaches to remain on track as you can see physical changes or feel the distinction in yourself. Get a kick out of the chance to take estimations and advance photographs every week or fortnight. Along these lines, be ready to track how far you have come and rolled out im-provements if fundamental. It keeps you responsible. It's a decent method to perceive how more grounded and speedier you are getting. Keep details. There's your weight, clearly, yet don't simply depend on the scales to demon-strate to you how far you've come. Record to what extent it took you to run your first mile, your initial 5K, whatever. In the event that it has a number, and you are hoping to enhance it, record it some way or another. Indeed, seeing numbers drop on the scale is incredible, however, so is seeing num-bers tumble off the stopwatch and your belt gaps.

- PLAN, PLAN, PLAN… design your dinners, anticipate being dynamic… at any rate toward the start. It takes around a month and a half to make an-other propensity. Planning is critical. Plan for time for abstaining from food, workouts, work and different exercises. Compose an arrangement each Sunday for the week ahead to set yourself up for progress. On Sundays you may get a kick out of the chance to prep your suppers, and work out your preparation/movement plan. Along these lines you know your arrangement or new routines, you're responsible and it is less demanding, stick to it. Planning is everything, as the saying goes "If YOU Neglect TO PLAN, YOU Intend TO Fall flat"… it's actually with regards to your sustenance…. on the off chance that you don't set up your suppers and titbits, you will get ravenous and eat whatever comes in your grasp… and we don't need that, isn't that so?

- Find an activity program you will take after. It makes it less demanding, particularly in the event that you are simply beginning.

- Find an activity accomplice, some person who will keep you responsible.

- Set a day to set up some solid dinners to keep you on track. Prepare solid supper on Sundays. You might make Natural product FILLED Heated Cereal, cut up some crisp vegetables, toss something in my simmering pot, for example, SALSA CHICKEN.

- Don't ever skip breakfast.

- Set up here and now exercise objectives for yourself and prizes. Your objectives ought to be constantly quantifiable with a time allotment. For example, **Push-ups** (do the greatest number of as you can from your toes, at that point drop to your knees and do knee push-ups… till 1 minute is up, record your score). **Bouncing squats** (do the greatest number of hopping squats as you can, on the off chance that you can't do anymore, proceed just with standard squats till 1 minute is up). **Set a clock and perceive to what extent you can hold a plank for.** For instance, "I will have the capacity to perform 10 push ups from my toes by December 1st, 2018"... and in the event that you accomplish that objective, you can compensate yourself. Reward yourself with something you appreciate... possibly another nail clean or another exercise tank top.

• Be sure ready for disappointment. You wouldn't be great. This will be common when you eat an excessive amount of pizza at the football gathering or skip four exercises in succession. The critical thing here is to foresee these minutes, proceed onward from them, and set yourself back on the wagon. A couple of missed exercises won't delete your diligent work and a couple of thousand additional calories won't set the pounds back on. It will happen. I've been there. It's anything but difficult to feel frustrated with yourself and surrender, yet don't. You would prefer not to back pedal to the start.

A Trip To Fitness

There are so many objectives to benefit from in the trip to fitness. It's like going on a little adventure where you will be exposed to new things for the betterment of the body. You will learn to cultivate a new eating habit, a positive mindset and lifestyle, new social bonds, routines, possible adjustments to the current way of life and at the end of the day you end up developing self- confidence. Most importantly, the building of self-confidence depends on the self-will and determination of the individual. Fitness is all about building a personality. This personality starts from when you make the decision to stay fit and healthy by all means possible. In which case you are really in for a change for a surprise. A change in your meal, thoughts and mindset (go-getter/positive mindset to keep going no matter what), routines (adjusting to new workouts and avoiding some foods with high carbs) and actions.

Self-confidence is a state of mind that you hold about yourself that enables you to push ahead and accomplish your objectives. In which case, a self-confident individual has a general feeling of control of his/her own life and can do what he/she wishes and anticipates. Self-confidence matters a lot in your trip to fitness, If you can't work on your self-confidence, you are likely to give up on achieving your fitness goals and dreams.

Steps To Take To Work on Your Self Confidence

- Prepare yourself to know what you want.

- Be benevolent and liberal.

- Continuously have a positive mindset.

- Slaughter negative contemplations.

- Dress to look great dependably.

- Become acquainted with yourself.

- Make and Know your standards to live up to them.

- Act positively.

- Stand tall.

- Work on your efficiencies.

- Set a little objective pertaining to your life dependably and accomplish it.

- Change a little propensity.

- Create an exposure to gaining valuable information by reading good books.

- Get a bullet journal to document and follow up on your lists of to-dos.

- Smile effortlessly.

- Make time to exercise.

- Give Yourself Permission To Be In The Process, Take Risks and Make Mistakes.

- Accomplish a long-term goal on what you've been working a while on.

- Speak Well to Yourself.

- Request Help and Offer Your Help to Others

Building Your Self Confidence.

Constructive reasoning, training, learning and conversing with other individuals are generally valuable approaches to enhance or lift your certainty levels. Certainty originates from sentiments of prosperity, acknowledgement of your body and brain (self-confidence) and faith in your own capacity, abilities and experience.

Exercise Regularly

Regular exercise affects you certainly. Normal exercise discharges endorphins which thus associate with the sedative receptors in the cerebrum. This brings a sort of pleasurable perspective and thus, you'll see yourself in a more positive light. The main exposure to creating a better Self-confidence starts with exercise. You might wonder why this book single-handed "exercise". This is because exercise is a personal choice. It depends on the individual and how serious or not they intend to carry on with the improvement of their appearance. Which means if you are serious about the body you want, you will be willing to do what it takes. The daring attitude comes in, the "I CAN" factor is brought to reality. You find yourself striving for positivity to become that you are almost there. You have complete faith in yourself and what you do and not quitting no matter what. That is where the new You is born. When you are consistently doing this, signs of self-improvement physically will show forth as well as you will feel more propelled to act in ways that manufacture your strengths.

If you are willing to embark on this trip to fitness, you must look for effective ways to improve and build your self-confidence. Once that is achieved and you are willing to do what it takes then avoid the obvious obstacles, the sky is set to be your limit.

I trust you appreciated those tips and feel roused to set out on your new, more advantageous way of life.

I wasn't anybody exceptional. I don't have a past filled with marathoners in my parentage. So when I say, "In the event that I can do it, anybody can," you can believe it. All it takes is the genuine desire to need to change your life. Furthermore, you're there, or else you wouldn't read this. Once more, congrats; life is going to show signs of improvement.

I want you to enjoy all that life has to offer and absolutely never give up!!!!

Remain fit and healthy!!!!

About The Author

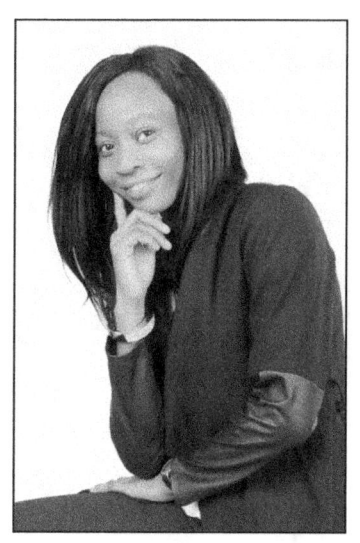

Beatrice Sargin is a certified Personal Trainer, Dancer, Microbiologist, Freelance Creative Ghost Writer and an Author. Her first book published was the Horrible Silence, an African tale. Her passions include writing, researching, arts, dancing, singing and travelling. She believes that when you work hard, you can achieve your prospective goals in due time. Trip to fitness is her 2nd published book.